Irritable Bowel Syndrome

Other books in this series:

Angina
Arthritis
Asthma
Bowel Cancer
Breast Cancer
Chronic Fatigue
Dementia
Depression
Diabetes
High Blood Pressure
How to Stay Healthy
How to Stop Smoking
Menopause
Osteoporosis

Coming soon:

Strokes

Irritable Bowel Syndrome

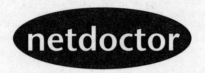

Series Editor
Dr Dan Rutherford
www.netdoctor.co.uk

Hodder & Stoughton
LONDON SYDNEY AUCKLAND

The material in this book is in no way intended to replace professional medical care or attention by a qualified practitioner. The materials in this book cannot and should not be used as a basis for diagnosis or choice of treatment.

Copyright © 2005 by NetDoctor.co.uk
Illustrations copyright © 2005 by Amanda Williams

First published in Great Britain in 2005

The right of NetDoctor.co.uk to be identified as the Author of the Work has been asserted by them in accordance with the Copyright, Designs and Patents Act 1988.

10 9 8 7 6 5 4 3 2 1

All rights reserved. No part of this publication may be reproduced, stored in a retrieval system, or transmitted, in any form or by any means, without the prior written permission of the publisher, nor be otherwise circulated in any form of binding or cover other than that in which it is published and without a similar condition being imposed on the subsequent purchaser.

British Library Cataloguing in Publication Data
A record for this book is available from the British Library

ISBN 0 340 86268 8

Typeset in Garamond by Avon DataSet Ltd, Bidford-on-Avon, Warwickshire

Printed and bound in Great Britain by Bookmarque Ltd, Croydon, Surrey

The paper and board used in this paperback are natural recyclable products made from wood grown in sustainable forests. The manufacturing processes conform to the environmental regulations of the country of origin.

Hodder & Stoughton
A Division of Hodder Headline Ltd
338 Euston Road
London NW1 3BH
www.madaboutbooks.com

Contents

	Foreword	ix
	Acknowledgements	xi
1	**What Is Irritable Bowel Syndrome?**	1
	Main symptoms of IBS	2
	IBS symptoms in practice	4
	Care in diagnosis	6
	Size of the problem	8
	Long-term nature	9
2	**The Bowel – What It Is and How It Works**	11
	The digestive system	11
	Structure of the gut	14
	Propulsion	16
	Muscle types	18
	Control of gut muscle	19
	Hormones acting on the gut	21
3	**Possible Causes of IBS**	24
	Inflammation of the gut	25
	Abnormal gut bacteria	26
	Oversensitivity of the gut	27
	Changes in 'gut-brain interaction'	27
	Disturbance of gut muscle action	28
	Food intolerance and allergy	29
	Genes	30
	Psychological factors	31
	'Functional' vs. 'physical' illness	33

4	**Tests**	34
	Why test?	35
	1. Age of the patient	36
	2. Presence of red flag symptoms	36
	3. Patient factors	43
	4. Predominance of diarrhoea	44
5	**Treatment for IBS**	50
	Is any treatment necessary?	50
	Are there other non-bowel related issues?	51
	Becoming informed about IBS	51
	Having realistic expectations	51
	General recommendations	52
	Your IBS 'type'	52
	Treating diarrhoea-predominant IBS	53
	Treating constipation-predominant IBS	57
	Treating abdominal pain and bloating	60
	Psychological therapy	63
6	**Complementary Medicine for IBS**	64
	Hypnotherapy	65
	Chinese herbal medicines	66
	Padma lax	66
	Artichoke leaf extract	67
	Probiotics	67
	Other complementary medicines	68
7	**Food Intolerance, Allergy and IBS**	69
	General immune system reactions	69
	IBS and allergy	70
	Food intolerance	71
	Elimination diets	72
	Conclusions	74

Appendix A: References	76
Appendix B: Medication for IBS	78
Appendix C: Useful Contacts	83

Foreword

Irritable bowel syndrome affects many of us at some time in our lives. Bowel upset, bloating and abdominal cramps can occur during periods of emotional stress; something well known to anybody sitting an exam! For the majority of people this is a temporary nuisance and does not warrant any form of medical or alternative intervention. For a significant proportion of the population, however, irritable bowel syndrome is more troublesome and has a significant impact upon the quality of life. Worries concerning the possible cause of abdominal symptoms – in particular a fear that symptoms are due to cancer – exacerbate the problem.

There is enormous press interest in irritable bowel syndrome – women's magazines, daily newspapers, radio and television often feature the condition. Unfortunately not all the information presented in the press has a strong evidence base and sometimes what is said is misleading and may increase, rather than lessen, anxiety. Fallacies concerning 'food allergy', candida infection of the gut and the use of specific diets are widespread; these do not help the desperate patient who is trying to help him or herself and some of the recommendations are potentially harmful.

This short book, written by an experienced medical practitioner, is particularly welcome because it is strongly evidence-based. The causes, investigation (when necessary) and treatment options are very clearly presented. There are sections devoted to 'alternative' therapies including hypnotherapy and dietary manipulations, allowing readers to reach their own conclusions about the full range of available treatment options – in a balanced and well-informed way.

The use of self-help books is to be greatly welcomed. The best ones inform without causing alarm, they point out sensible approaches to treatment and help us avoid cranky, illogical therapies which lack evidence for efficacy. This is an extremely good self-help book.

> Dr Kelvin R. Palmer MD, FRCP(Ed), FRCP(Lond), FRCS(Ed)
> Consultant Gastroenterologist
> Western General Hospital, Edinburgh

Acknowledgements

Each of the books in this series attempts to provide the lay reader with a digest of information on an important medical topic. The information aims to be as up-to-date as possible. Dr Kelvin Palmer, Consultant Gastroenterologist at the Western General Hospital in Edinburgh, kindly ensured that my facts were both correct and contemporary. I thank him sincerely for taking the time to do this on top of his already busy work schedule.

As ever I am also indebted to the teams at Hodder and at home who ensure that each of these short books is produced as near to the promised deadline as possible ...

Comments on the content of this book are welcome, whether they be concerning mistakes (hopefully few) or of improvements that can make the information more helpful. You can email me at dan.rutherford@netdoctor.co.uk by putting 'Hodder' in the subject line.

Dr Dan Rutherford BSc, MB, ChB, MRCGP, FRCP(Edin)
Medical Director
www.netdoctor.co.uk

Chapter 1

What Is Irritable Bowel Syndrome?

The internal workings of the human body are almost entirely automatic. We don't have to consciously breathe in and out, or choose the rate of our heartbeat. We control our body temperature and blood pressure very accurately but without giving either a thought, and the digestive system gets on with the job of extracting energy from food and eliminating waste according to its own agenda. The only conscious input we normally have to the latter process is to decide what sorts of food we'll eat in the first place. Even responding to the calls of nature that result is something we can only partly influence deliberately.

In irritable bowel syndrome the digestive system comes out of the background and makes its presence obvious. The impact of irritable bowel syndrome – IBS to those who know it – can vary from mildly troublesome to a major interference with daily life. The precise symptoms that IBS causes can vary between individuals and even from day to day in one person, but there are common themes among them.

Main symptoms of IBS

Irritable bowel syndrome is not a new disorder. It is well described in medical texts from at least the nineteenth century, although in those days it did not have the modern name. Most of the medical attention that IBS has received has, however, occurred in the past 25 years, as doctors have recognised that a cluster of symptoms concerned with the function of the digestive system affects very large numbers of people. These common symptoms include:

- Abdominal discomfort or pain that is related to moving the bowel. Often people feel 'bloated'.
- Alterations in the frequency and consistency of the stools – diarrhoea or constipation or a combination of the two.

These are the core symptoms of IBS but there are many others. Over recent years medical experts have collaborated to agree a set of criteria that more accurately define what IBS is. As these have evolved out of meetings held in Rome they are called the 'Rome criteria' and they are now in their second version:

'ROME II' CRITERIA FOR IBS

Within the past 12 months there have been at least 3 months (not necessarily consecutive) in which abdominal pain or discomfort has been present and which has at least two of the following features:

- The pain is relieved by opening the bowels.
- There is also a change in the frequency of the stool.
- There is also a change in the appearance of the stool.

It is an essential part of the diagnosis of IBS that no other abnormality is found to explain the symptoms. We'll come back in detail to this issue but one of the mysteries of IBS is that it occurs in the absence of anything obviously 'wrong' with the bowel. In other words, in IBS ordinary medical tests on the bowel are normal.

The Rome criteria also refer to other symptoms that often occur in IBS:

- Problems with passing the stool (for example a need to strain, a feeling of incomplete emptying or of urgency, in which people get a sudden need to go to the toilet).
- Bloating of the tummy. It is often noted by people with IBS that even in the course of a single day they will feel the need to loosen their clothing or slacken their belt to cope with this feeling.
- Stools may be changed in form (lumpy, hard, watery or loose).
- Stools may be changed in frequency (more than three per day or fewer than three per week).
- Mucus may be passed with or separately from the stools.

IBS symptoms in practice

Symptom lists determined by international committees of medical experts have their uses but in practice the variety of symptoms that IBS can be associated with is very much more varied. The Rome criteria constitute the main symptoms but there can be plenty of others on top. Irritable bowel syndrome may occur at almost any age but most commonly starts in the late teenage years or early adulthood. The source of the symptoms is mainly the digestive system, although in the next chapter we look at how other factors are also involved.

The part of the digestive system most often affected is the lower bowel, but not exclusively so. Other areas of the digestive system can also be affected by IBS, in which case the symptom patterns vary respectively. They can also vary over time in the same person. For example, IBS can arise (or is presumed to arise) in the:

GULLET (OESOPHAGUS)
- This can give rise to a sensation like a golf ball in the throat between meals which does not interfere with swallowing (called 'globus').
- Painful swallowing but without hold-up of food. (When food does get held up on the way down this can indicate a more serious cause, although IBS, rarely, can cause this too.)

STOMACH
- This can cause discomfort very much like that of an ulcer in the stomach or in the immediate outlet of the stomach (duodenum), yet on investigation no ulcer is found. This is called 'non-ulcer dyspepsia'.
- Feeling full after small meals. This may reach the stage of not being able to finish a meal.
- Abdominal bloating after meals.

UPPER BOWEL (ALSO CALLED THE 'SMALL BOWEL' – SEE CHAPTER 2)
- Increased gurgling noises, which may be loud enough to cause social embarrassment (the medical term for such noises is particularly apt – 'borborygmi').
- Abdominal bloating, which may be so severe that a woman may describe herself as looking pregnant. Bloating usually subsides overnight and returns the following day.
- Generalised abdominal tenderness, associated with bloating.

LOWER BOWEL (ALSO CALLED THE 'LARGE BOWEL')
- Right-sided abdominal pain, either low or tucked up under the right ribs. This may or may not get better on opening the bowels.
- Pain tucked up under the left ribs. When this pain is bad enough, it may even be felt in the left armpit.
- Variable and erratic bowel habits alternating from constipation to diarrhoea. An urgent need to empty the bowel can be the most disabling symptom of IBS. It can be bad enough to cause incontinence in some people.
- Increased gastro-colic reflex (see page 20).

- Severe, short stabbing pains in the rectum, called 'proctalgia fugax'.

OTHER SYMPTOMS
- Headaches
- In women, left-sided abdominal pain during intercourse
- Passing urine more often
- Fatigue and tiredness
- Sleep disturbance
- Loss of appetite
- Nausea
- Anxiety, depression and stress-related symptoms, which may interact with gut symptoms

Care in diagnosis

None of the symptoms referred to above is exclusive to IBS. Similar symptoms, and combinations of symptoms, can occur with a host of other conditions affecting the bowel, including the most serious ones such as bowel cancer. The range of possible causes for many of the non-bowel symptoms such as headache, urinary frequency and fatigue are of course even wider.

Like any important medical condition it is essential that irritable bowel syndrome is properly and confidently diagnosed and yet, as we've just seen, it is a condition that can take many guises. Although it is very often possible for a doctor to make a diagnosis of IBS with a high degree of confidence just by listening to the patient's history, it will often be necessary to go through a range of medical tests to be sure. (These tests are outlined in chapter 4.) Not everyone needs the full battery of tests – young adults especially may need only a few because they so rarely have one of the serious bowel conditions – but this is a decision that the doctor needs to make in partnership with the patient on an individual basis.

Some symptoms are most definitely *not* due to irritable bowel syndrome and if they are present then a hunt for the correct explanation is essential. Often these are called 'red flag' symptoms for obvious reasons. Examples of red flag symptoms in connection with the digestive system are:

- Weight loss
- Passage of blood from the back passage
- New onset of symptoms in an older adult (over 40)
- Symptoms awakening the patient from sleep (although the pain of IBS can do this, it is unusual to have night-time diarrhoea)
- Anaemia (bloodlessness) or some other abnormality on blood tests
- Persistent diarrhoea or severe constipation (IBS tends to cause intermittent symptoms)
- Recurrent sticking of food on swallowing
- Vomiting
- Family history of bowel cancer or one of the conditions that inflames the bowel (such as Crohn's disease or ulcerative colitis – see page 48)

The above is not an exhaustive list but the point is that IBS is not a diagnosis that one should rush at without due care. Nor is it a diagnosis you can make yourself. Certainly a red flag symptom must be investigated thoroughly but anyone who has *any* of the symptoms referred to above should see a doctor about them.

Size of the problem

IBS is by far the commonest cause of recurrent abdominal symptoms in adults and adolescents. Studies throughout the world have shown that it affects between 10 and 20 per cent of the population, of whom only a minority consult a doctor about it. IBS occurs in people over 70 with about the same frequency as in younger adults, although these are largely people who have had IBS in their younger years and have taken it with them into older age. IBS as a new condition is rare in the elderly.

Although GPs deal with the majority of people who come to them with IBS, a substantial proportion of patients are referred to specialists to have the diagnosis confirmed or for treatment advice. IBS is consequently the commonest condition that specialists in digestive diseases see and as so many of the people referred go on to have additional tests it is a condition that consumes vast amounts of medical resource.

IBS is not 'serious' in the same way that bowel cancer is serious – people with IBS live as long as anyone else – but they can be badly affected by it and it can cause a great deal of ill health and absence from work. For a condition that is so difficult to understand, for which the cause is unknown and in which the bowel is apparently 'normal', it causes a huge amount of trouble.

WORLD-WIDE PROBLEM
One of the particularly interesting aspects of IBS is that it is about equally common across the world. This contrasts with some other important bowel conditions such as bowel cancer

and diverticulitis, which are generally more common in Western society. As we think that dietary differences, such as a lack of roughage in the Western diet, are important factors in causing the regional variations in the latter conditions, the fact that IBS crosses borders so easily suggests that diet is not such an important factor in its development. This observation is also borne out when coming to treat IBS (chapter 5) as increasing dietary roughage benefits only a proportion of people with the condition.

GENDER DIFFERENCE
Population surveys show that women experience IBS symptoms about twice as commonly as do men. In the UK proportionately more women than men consult their GP about the symptoms, so the view from the GP's surgery is even more that IBS is mainly a female problem. Why this should be is, however, not well explained within the various theories that we have about the possible causes of IBS. Sometimes IBS develops in a woman following removal of her uterus (hysterectomy), particularly if she has a history of multiple or difficult births. This may be due to nerve damage within the pelvis due to the operation.

Long-term nature

IBS does not tend to go away. Over three quarters of people who develop IBS will still have symptoms several years later and many people remain susceptible to IBS throughout their adult lives. It does, however, tend to wax and wane, so bad spells of a few weeks may be followed by good spells that are as long or longer. Sometimes exacerbations of IBS are related to stressful life events such as relationship problems, work stress or other identifiable reasons. Most of the time no such obvious factors can be blamed.

Both to the people who have the condition and to the health personnel who have to care for them IBS is a major health issue. Before we go much further in considering what theories we have about causes, as well as the available treatments, we should cover in a bit more detail what is meant by the 'bowel', how it works and what seems to go wrong with it in IBS.

Chapter 2

The Bowel – What It Is and How It Works

The digestive system

The digestive system (also called the digestive tract) is in effect a long tube starting at the mouth and finishing at the anus, which along its length is divided into areas with different functions (figure 1).

UPPER DIGESTIVE SYSTEM
The upper part of the digestive system consists of:

- The mouth, along with the teeth, tongue and salivary glands
- The gullet (oesophagus) – the tube that conducts food from the mouth, through the middle of the chest to the stomach
- The stomach. Here the digestive tube widens out to form a reservoir in which food is mixed with acid and enzymes to break it down further

Figure 1: Diagram of the digestive tract

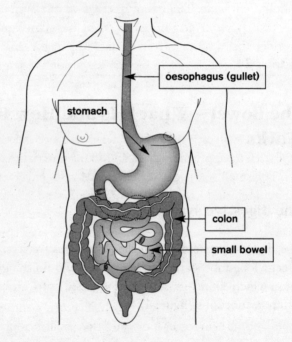

MIDDLE TO LOWER DIGESTIVE SYSTEM

From the opening of the stomach, all the way to the anus, is the bowel, or 'gut'. This is divided into two regions with different structure and function. The first part is the 'small bowel', so named because it is narrower than the 'large bowel'. It is about 3cm wide and is between 4 metres and 7 metres long in adults. The lining of the small bowel is specialised to absorb the nutrients that we need from food, which by the time it reaches this part of the digestive tract is a mushy liquid. Indigestible elements in food, such as fibre, along with any unabsorbed liquids continue down the small bowel and pass into the large bowel.

The large bowel is shorter, at about 1.25 metres, but is about 7cm wide. The main function of the large bowel is to extract water and minerals from the semi-liquid food residue that reaches it from the last part of the small bowel. As food waste travels along the length of the large bowel it therefore becomes drier and firmer, eventually becoming formed stool.

The lower part of the large bowel, called the rectum, acts as a reservoir for stool. Periodically we become aware of the need to empty the rectum and so the process is complete.

The small and large bowel regions respectively make up the middle and lower sections of the digestive system. An alternative term for the large bowel is the 'colon' and until fairly recently irritable bowel syndrome was commonly called 'irritable colon', 'spastic colon' or even 'mucous colitis', all of these terms suggesting that disturbed function of the large bowel alone was the source of the trouble. As we'll see later, IBS is more complex than this and also involves not only the small bowel but the brain, the nervous system and the effects of various hormones on the digestive system. The term 'irritable bowel syndrome' hardly does justice to the diverse nature of the problem.

Although it is convenient to describe the digestive tract as a series of sections, it is of course all one continuous system. To work properly all the regions somehow need to co-ordinate their actions. This aspect is worth looking at, as it is here that IBS seems to have its cause.

Structure of the gut

If you were to take a typical part of the small bowel, cut it across and examine it in detail you would see several structures that are represented in diagrammatic form in figure 2. Going from the inside out:

Figure 2: Cross-section of the gut

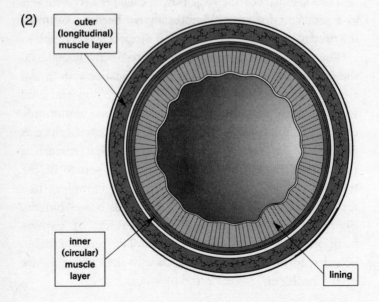

1. LINING

The precise details of the inner lining vary according to which part of the gut you are looking at. In the upper small bowel the lining is folded to increase its surface area, which makes it more efficient at absorbing nutrients from food. In figure 2 the section is from lower down in the small bowel, where the lining has smoothed out a bit.

2. MUSCLE LAYERS

The next main layer is comprised of muscle, but this is divided into two layers. The inner muscle layer runs in a

Figure 3: Contraction of circular gut muscle

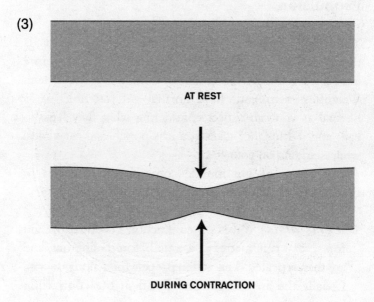

circle around the wall of the bowel. Contraction of these muscle fibres narrows the bowel at the point of contraction, squeezing the contents of the bowel and increasing the pressure within the bowel (figure 3).

Outside the circular muscle layer lies the longitudinal muscle layer, in which the fibres run along the line of the bowel. Contraction of these muscle fibres shortens the length of the bowel at the point of contraction (figure 4a).

3. NERVES AND BLOOD VESSELS

Scattered throughout the wall of the bowel are the blood vessels that take blood to and from the gut as well as an extensive network of nerve fibres, linking up all the muscle fibres.

Propulsion

The whole digestive tract from the gullet onwards is therefore one long tube of muscle. Gravity is therefore unnecessary for the movement of food along the system. Weightless astronauts have normal gut function (or as normal as you can expect considering what they have to eat!) and if the fancy takes you it is possible to eat a meal while standing on your head.

The layers of gut muscle combine their actions to produce two main contraction patterns of the gut:

1 **'Peristalsis'**: Waves of contraction go down the gut for several centimetres at a time before fading out, and are then repeated. This action propels food along the gut. Usually the area of gut just ahead of the contraction

Figure 4a: Contraction of longitudinal gut muscle

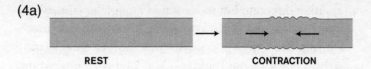

Figure 4b: Peristalsis

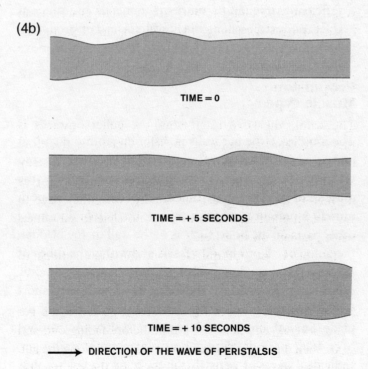

relaxes and widens, and this too travels along with the contraction wave (figure 4b). Waves of peristalsis can go in either direction but those waves that go 'upstream', i.e. which propel food back towards the mouth, are much shorter lived than the waves that propel food downstream, towards the anus. It is still a bit of mystery how the gut ensures this happens but it is under the control of the nerves that run extensively through the length of the gut.

2 ***Mixing movements***: The other main result of muscle action in the gut is to churn food up. This ensures even mixing of food with the digestive enzymes and the most efficient extraction of nutrients, minerals and water at the various stages along the bowel. Instead of producing movement in one direction these mixing actions move the food to and fro.

Muscle types

The muscle of the gut walls is different from the type of muscle we have that moves our limbs. Without getting too technical the gut contains 'smooth muscle' whereas the muscles of movement are called 'skeletal muscle'. Smooth muscle is present not just in the gut but is found in many other parts of the body, such as in the wall of the bladder, the lining of all our blood vessels and within the tubes of the airways in the lungs. Skeletal muscles are commonly called upon to contract and relax again in a very short period of time – say to move the fingers in playing the piano. Smooth muscle is more tuned to slow contractions over long periods lasting hours at a time, or longer. Individual waves of peristalsis in the gut last a few seconds at a time and are fairly rapid but in general gut muscle moves at a slow pace compared to skeletal muscle.

The smooth muscle of the gut may be a bit slow, but it is not weak. Waves of pressure generated by the gut muscles during normal bowel activity propel food and stools along, but usually the amount of pressure is not very great. Most people who do not have IBS are unaware of this activity. Overactivity of the gut muscle is one of the probable ways in which IBS occurs, when the increased pressure that results becomes all too obvious.

Control of gut muscle

Skeletal muscle is largely under conscious command whereas smooth muscle action, including that of the gut, is not. Gut muscle action is, however, highly organised and regulated by two systems:

1 Nerves within the gut wall
2 Hormones acting on the gut

GUT NERVOUS SYSTEM
The nervous system of the bowel is very complex – there are as many nerve cells within the walls of the digestive system as there are within the whole spinal cord. Its function is largely to control the muscle actions that go on.

Peristalsis and the mixing of food are reflex actions: muscle activity that happens automatically as a result of the way the gut nerves are 'wired' to each other. The signals that control these actions travel to and fro along the nerves within the gut wall. However, the gut is also connected by a great many nerves to the spinal cord and ultimately also to the brain. Arising from these more complex connections are other reflexes, some of which are perhaps familiar. For example, most people are aware that at times the urge to empty the bowel can be triggered by eating. Most commonly this occurs in the morning after breakfast. It is not just force of habit or convenience that is responsible, it is a recognised reflex action, called the 'gastro-colic reflex' (*gastro* – stomach and *colic* – colon). In this reflex the filling of the stomach with food triggers activity in certain nerve cells that send signals down the gut to the muscles that cause the bowel to empty. There are other similarly 'long-range' reflexes within the gut and although it is not important to know about them in detail it is useful to appreciate that they exist.

Anyone who has experienced the effects of emotion upon their bowel function knows also that the brain is intimately connected to the digestive system. Exam nerves or other causes of anxiety usually precipitate increased gut activity and often lead to diarrhoea. However, the brain has only a background role in the overall control of the digestive system – the gut's internal nervous system has the dominant effects.

NERVE SIGNALLING
One other piece of theory can be filed away at this stage but is useful later when looking at how drugs for IBS work. It concerns the way in which nerve signals are passed between nerve cells and to the muscles within the gut wall. Although it is useful to think of nerves as a bit like electrical cables and for nerve signals to be like electricity travelling

down the wires, this is not a very accurate description of what actually happens in living tissue. Nerve cells and fibres are extremely small and their junctions with each other are even smaller, but if you were to examine the junction between two nerves or between a nerve and a muscle, you would see that they do not actually touch. Instead, at these points there is a highly specialised zone called the synapse, at which the two nerves (or the nerve and the muscle) come very close but a small gap remains between them. Instead of a pulse of electricity what actually flows across this gap are tiny amounts of chemicals called neurotransmitters.

Tiny 'packets' of neurotransmitter substances are manufactured by nerve cells and are held in readiness at the synapses. A signal travelling down the first nerve triggers the release of some neurotransmitters from its ending, which travel across the gap and attach to the next nerve, or muscle. This action triggers a reaction from the nerve or muscle, and so the signal is passed on. The process is illustrated in figure 5.

The body uses a range of neurotransmitter substances, about which quite a lot is now known. Researchers have as a result been able to design drug treatments based on blocking or enhancing their effects. This forms the basis of some of the treatments used for IBS (as well as a great many other medical conditions) and we'll return to this topic in chapter 5.

Hormones acting on the gut

A hormone is a natural chemical substance produced in one part of the body but which has some sort of action on another part of the body. It reaches its 'target' via the

Figure 5: Junction between nerve cells (synapse) showing the way signals are passed from cell to cell

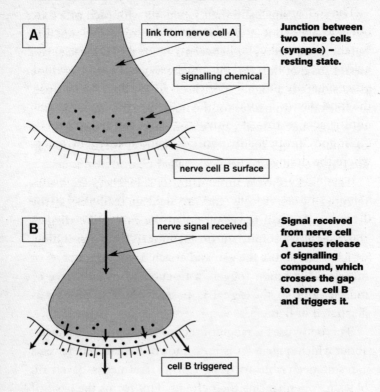

bloodstream. In several regions of the digestive system, notably the stomach and upper part of the small bowel, the presence of digested food causes the release of hormones from special cells within the lining of the gut. These are transported via the blood supply to another part of the gut and can influence its activity. For example, the arrival of stomach acid into the upper small bowel causes the release of a hormone called secretin. Secretin slows down the action of the gut in general. This has a regulating effect on the release of more food from the stomach.

The co-ordinated actions of the nerves and the hormones of the gut therefore provide the controls needed for this long and complicated structure to work. Food is held in the stomach and released slowly once the acids and other digestive juices have broken down food initially. As the food travels down the gut it is again mixed and digested until it gets to the stage that nutrients can be absorbed. On it goes, propelled by peristalsis, and reaches the colon where the drying out process occurs.

It should be evident by now that digestion is by no means a simple process that follows as food is simply shunted along the gut. Like anything complex there is plenty of scope for things going wrong. Summarising present theories on what goes wrong in IBS is what we cover next.

Chapter 3

Possible Causes of IBS

We said earlier there is no known cause for IBS. Although true, that should not be taken to mean that we have no ideas. There are many plausible theories of the cause, or causes, of IBS. If one looks at the many symptoms that can occur in IBS, from diarrhoea to constipation or combinations of both, as well as the many others, it makes sense that no single explanation would be likely to cover everything. Irritable bowel syndrome is a convenient catch-all term but it is not likely to be just one condition.

Inflammation of the gut

'Inflammation' means the body's response to injury and the sort of injury that might be relevant to irritable bowel syndrome is gut infection. About 25 per cent of people with IBS can date the onset of their symptoms to an episode of diarrhoea and vomiting (gastroenteritis) that they had months or years before and which would be likely to have been caused by infection. Follow-up surveys of people who have had gastroenteritis due to a confirmed gut infection show they are much more likely than the average population to get IBS symptoms in the months afterwards. No one bug is particularly likely to cause IBS symptoms later, except to say that bacterial infections of the gut are more likely to do so than virus infections, which in the UK are the commoner. Most gastroenteritis episodes are brief – a few days to a week long – but if the illness is prolonged then later IBS symptoms are more likely.

Exactly what a gut infection may do to the bowel that can lead to IBS is not known. Detailed analysis of the bowel lining does not show any consistent abnormalities. It is possible, though, that the infection causes subtle damage to the gut nervous system that is hard to detect but fails to recover.

Of course if someone who has an episode of gastroenteritis, especially if it is following a trip to a country where food poisoning is a regular risk, goes on having the symptoms afterwards, tests need to be done to ensure that the infection has in fact cleared up. Some types of gut infection can persist for months or years afterwards. Tests to ensure that persistent infection is ruled out would be necessary in someone with IBS symptoms who had a history of travel exposure.

Gut infection is an attractive explanation for IBS but it cannot be the main one. 75 per cent of people with IBS have no prior history of gastroenteritis and most people who get gastroenteritis do not subsequently get IBS.

Abnormal gut bacteria

The contents of the upper digestive system are normally almost free of bacteria – few bugs can survive in the acidic environment of the stomach. The small bowel in healthy people contains small numbers of bacteria such as *lactobacilli* – the bacteria that cause milk to go sour. The large bowel (colon) is quite different and normally contains high numbers of bacteria of many different types. Normally we live in harmony with these bacteria, which appear to provide several benefits to their hosts. For example, because of their high numbers the normal bacterial population of the large bowel provides too much competition for harmful bacteria to easily get a hold. Gut bacteria also produce vitamin K and other vitamins of the B group that are useful to us.

Alterations to the gut bacterial populations are a possible cause of IBS. A reduction in flatulence and abdominal pain was seen in a study that boosted the amounts of *lactobacilli* in the gut of people with IBS. There is much current research interest in using probiotics – dietary supplements containing 'helpful' bacteria as a treatment for IBS. (The advertising industry has also got hold of these supplements in a big way recently and all sorts of health improvements are *claimed* to flow from using them.)

Oversensitivity of the gut

Research in the 1970s looked at whether people with IBS were unduly sensitive to normal gut activity. This could come about in two ways – either the gut in IBS was unduly sensitive and was sending out pain signals too easily, or the person with IBS becomes too aware of otherwise normal sensations. Or both could be happening.

The digestive system is continuously active but most of the time we are unaware of it. If people with IBS have a low 'pain threshold' for gut activity then they would experience symptoms that others would not notice. This is a difficult theory to test and the main method has been to inflate a small balloon inserted into some part of the digestive tract (originally it was the lower bowel or rectum) and record the pressure at which the subject becomes uncomfortable. 60 per cent of people with IBS had discomfort at lower pressures than average but the experimental technique had some influence. If the pressures were steadily increased then the IBS subjects had a lower threshold for noticing discomfort. If the pressures were varied randomly then there was no difference from the average. This could mean that people with IBS become sensitised to their symptoms and each time the sequence of abdominal pain and bowel disturbance starts they are already anticipating what will happen next, thus reinforcing the symptoms.

Changes in 'gut-brain interaction'

This is really an expansion of the previous concept that the person with IBS has developed an over-sensitive gut or notices normal gut activity too easily. The link between the brain and the digestive system has already been mentioned and it is usually a background process. Recent brain scanning techniques have made it possible to detect which parts of the brain are most active at any one time. Some people with IBS show brain activity in different areas to non-IBS subjects when both are subjected to gut stimulation such as balloon inflation.

If there is some mileage in these theories of increased gut sensitivity, lowered pain thresholds or alterations in the way that the brain and the gut communicate with each other, we are far from easily putting it all together. Somewhere in there may be the explanation for IBS, but for what percentage of sufferers is presently unknown.

Disturbance of gut muscle action

This is one of the earliest theories of the cause of IBS. Gut muscle, as we mentioned in the last chapter, shows the ability to contract in purposeful ways, either to propel food along (peristalsis) or mix it up. This ability is built in to the gut's design, you could say, and a piece of gut removed at operation will still show this activity for as long as it remains alive. IBS would nicely be explained if the inbuilt activity of gut muscle changed. People with IBS who tend to get diarrhoea rather than constipation do tend to show a shortened time that it takes for food eaten to arrive at the anus (this is called the transit time) but transit time varies a lot in healthy individuals anyway and it is impossible to know if a change in transit time is a cause or a consequence of IBS.

Food intolerance and allergy

Depending on how you define 'food intolerance' you could say that we all have this to some degree. Very few people could eat anything and never have a problem with it. It is no surprise, therefore, that many people with IBS notice that some foods trigger their symptoms or make them feel worse. Although there is no doubting the existence of food intolerance, the term is also much abused, as is 'food allergy' (perhaps more so).

Food *intolerance* implies that some foods are associated with symptoms but that usually one needs to take at least a minimum amount of this food for it to have an effect. Smaller amounts of the same food are tolerable. Food *allergy* implies that even small amounts of the food can trigger symptoms.

True food allergy is rare. In food allergy removal of the offending item from the diet should prevent the symptoms from occurring, the challenge being to detect what the problem food may be. This may be difficult if the person is particularly sensitive to small amounts. Food intolerance is easier to detect as a recognisable amount of the food is required to cause symptoms. Coeliac disease, an allergic reaction of the gut to gluten (a protein present in certain cereals), is an important cause of IBS-like symptoms. It is discussed further in Chapter 4 (page 46).

Many studies on dietary adjustment in people with IBS show a positive effect. This is at least partly due to the 'placebo effect'. A placebo is an inert or 'dummy' treatment which when tested still shows positive results. The placebo effect always needs to be taken into account when evaluating any type of medical treatment, and is often found to be powerfully present in treatments for IBS. The basic tool is the exclusion diet, in which someone goes on to a very limited range of foods and then slowly introduces more items until symptoms start to appear. A quick search on the Internet will reveal any number of outlets purporting to help detect your food 'allergies'. The majority of these are based on shaky science or none at all and do-it-yourself diagnosis of this sort is usually not a good idea. It can at least be misleading and could potentially be dangerous if it causes delay in a correct diagnosis. On the other hand, allergic conditions tend to get less attention than they deserve from conventional medicine. A summary of what you can reasonably do to detect and deal with food intolerance and allergy is in chapter 7.

Genes

An individual's risk of getting almost any illness is now seen as the outcome of their genetic tendency towards that condition combined with their exposure in life to some factor that will bring the illness to the surface. Certainly this seems to hold true of many major diseases such as diabetes, high blood pressure, asthma, many types of cancer, arthritis – the list is a long one – but the extent of any genetic link in IBS is uncertain. As IBS is more common in identical twins than in non-identical twins this gives support to genes having some effect, but there is certainly no particular gene 'type' associated with the condition.

There are probably many possible trigger factors but we know very little about what they may be. Gut infection looks as though it is one of them. Stress is probably another.

Psychological factors

People who have IBS commonly report that stress makes their symptoms worse. Surveys of people with IBS who attend specialist clinics for the condition show that they are more likely to have psychological conditions in addition, such as depression and/or anxiety. The link between emotional factors and bowel function is not in doubt but the relationship between IBS and psychological illness is complicated and often misunderstood. A number of important issues need to be borne in mind in this important area.

MIND VS. BODY
Western medicine tends to split illnesses into those considered 'physical' and others considered 'psychological'. Such split thinking has lots of disadvantages and it is increasingly recognised by the health professions that one needs instead to consider the whole person. 'Holistic' medicine has always been part of the methodology of the most effective doctors but it will be a long time before it is the norm.

No illness is wholly one or the other. 'Physical' illness always has a psychological side, which may have very important effects on how one person's illness behaves. Psychological illness always impacts to some extent on the function of the body. Illnesses in which a physical cause cannot be found to explain the symptoms are called 'functional' illnesses. This is meant to convey that the 'fault' lies not in the components of the machinery of the human body but in the way they work together. Irritable bowel syndrome is considered to be a 'functional bowel disorder'.

ATTITUDES TO PSYCHOLOGICAL ASPECTS OF ILLNESS

Many doctors feel a lot less secure dealing with functional conditions compared to those for which the cause can be shown on a blood test, scan or X-ray. In IBS all the tests are normal – how then can you explain to the patient who has all the symptoms that there is 'nothing wrong'? Far from being taken as good news that no very serious condition has been revealed these negative test results can be deflating. People with IBS know they have a real problem and may be frustrated that the doctor doesn't seem able to give an adequate reason for it. General practitioners deal with the majority of patients with IBS but they have little formal training in the management of psychological conditions and are always under a great deal of time pressure. Thus we have this bias towards treating all medical problems with drugs, which tends to be quicker and easier to do, and hardly touching the psychological side.

However, the problems associated with the psychological aspects of illness run deeper than the practical ones of pressurised consultation time and the under-availability of psychologists. There is a stigma attached to psychological illness. To many people psychological (or functional) conditions get labelled as 'all in the mind', which is tantamount to saying they are imaginary. Irritable bowel syndrome suffers to some extent from this narrow-minded thinking, yet anyone with IBS knows only too well that their symptoms are very real.

Getting the balance right between the physical and psychological aspects of any illness is difficult for both the patients and the doctors. Surveys of general practitioners' views of the management of IBS show that the patients they have the most difficulty treating are those who are the least likely to accept that they could have any psychological problems. This fits with what we already know – most people are reluctant to be told that they have a psychological condition and are more comfortable with a physical explanation for what's wrong with them.

'Functional' vs. 'physical' illness

IBS is only one of many so-called functional illnesses. Others include chronic fatigue, fibromyalgia, unexplained headaches and some types of abdominal pain. In fact, people with IBS are more likely to suffer from one or more of these other conditions as well. Present medical knowledge finds it difficult to explain these conditions, compared to, say, something as obvious as a broken bone. Yet a little bit of digging shows that our knowledge of the fundamental processes behind all illness is quite shallow. Taking this example further it appears superficially that we understand how to fix a broken bone by setting it in a certain way in plaster for so many weeks, and so on. Yet we have no idea what processes switch on the bone-manufacturing cells or how it is that they 'know' how to rejoin the two ends of the break. Once you start asking more probing questions you realise that uncertainty is normal in explaining disease processes – it is only a question of degree.

Functional illness is therefore no different from any other, except that the degree of uncertainty about causes is relatively high. Research has yet to catch up with IBS and we can't wait that long before trying to treat it. The psychological aspect of IBS is important, as it is in all illness.

Chapter 4

Tests

There is no test that, if positive, says that you have irritable bowel syndrome. Instead IBS is diagnosed when it is clear that there is no other detectable cause for the symptoms experienced. It is a 'diagnosis of exclusion'. That might seem to imply that everyone who develops IBS symptoms for the first time needs to have all the tests under the sun and only if they are all negative can IBS be diagnosed with confidence.

Such a scattergun approach to testing would, however, be quite inappropriate. Not only would it involve exposing people to unnecessary investigation (and some of these tests are invasive to a degree) but it would place already stretched medical resources under avoidable extra strain. It would be too expensive and most importantly it is not what someone with IBS either needs or wants. In reality the majority of people with IBS can be positively identified without resort to any tests.

Why test?

One might therefore ask why do any tests at all on someone who seems likely to have IBS? Medical tests have many functions other than the obvious one of helping the doctor diagnose the condition. It is also reassuring to know that no 'serious' disease has been found. Confirming what the doctor thought in the first place increases confidence in the doctor and makes it more likely that his or her treatment will work. In other words tests can have a therapeutic value.

There are downsides to tests as well. They may reveal unwelcome or unexpected results, including findings of doubtful value. For example, gallstones might coincidentally be shown in the gallbladder but if they have caused no problems beforehand are they best ignored now? Most people's fear when they start to get abdominal symptoms is that they have something serious like bowel cancer. Sometimes investigation confirms their fears are justified.

The fundamental aim of the tests done in IBS is to detect other conditions that could cause the same symptoms. To ensure patients get the tests that they need (and avoid those that they do not) some filtering is required. There is no hard and fast way of doing this so the following is an example, based on four stages of filtering:

1. Age of the patient
2. Presence of 'red flag' symptoms
3. Patient factors
4. Predominance of diarrhoea

1. Age of the patient

Young adults are unlikely to have one of the more serious causes of abdominal symptoms, specifically bowel cancer. The age at which to set the cut-off is arbitrary but 40 is the general rule (some say 50, others 45). If someone younger than this has a history of symptoms that is typical for IBS and does not come into any of the other categories noted in the other three stages below then it is acceptable to make a diagnosis of IBS without going further. If the symptoms are of very recent onset then it is important for the doctor and patient to meet again a few times over the following few months to check that nothing else is happening (such as, for example, weight loss or anaemia) that should mean a rethink is in order.

2. Presence of red flag symptoms

These were mentioned in chapter 1. To recap, any of the following require full investigation:

- Weight loss
- Passage of blood from the back passage
- New onset of symptoms in an older adult (over 40)
- Symptoms awakening the patient from sleep (although the pain of IBS can do this, it is unusual to have night-time diarrhoea)
- Anaemia (bloodlessness) or some other abnormality on blood tests
- Persistent diarrhoea or severe constipation (IBS causes intermittent symptoms)
- Recurrent sticking of food on swallowing

- Vomiting
- Family history of bowel cancer or one of the conditions that inflames the bowel (such as Crohn's disease or ulcerative colitis – see page 48)

It is beyond the scope of this book to describe an exhaustive list of possible alternative diagnoses to IBS that could account for any or all of these red flag symptoms. Bowel cancer and inflammatory bowel disease are the main ones and are described in a bit more detail shortly. The tests that would be necessary to comprehensively check for these other conditions include:

HISTORY

A careful history is still the most important medical 'test' and is essential for revealing many of these features in the first place. The examination of the abdomen by the doctor is a part of good medical practice but usually does not reveal anything untoward in the majority of bowel problems, including IBS.

On the history side of things from the patient's point of view keeping a food diary for a few weeks can sometimes reveal problem foods that previously had not been suspected.

BLOOD TESTS

Simple blood tests are required in all people presenting for the first time with abdominal symptoms and these will be sufficient to detect anaemia or to suggest some types of vitamin deficiency. At the same time some other blood tests can be done in patients in whom diarrhoea is predominant (see page 53).

ENDOSCOPY

Endoscopy is the general name for optical inspection of the inside of the digestive system, using flexible fibre-optic instruments. These came to prominence in the 1970s and have been continuously refined along with the miniaturisation of sophisticated electronics and development of digital cameras. Endoscopes can be introduced through the mouth to inspect the upper digestive system down to the upper small bowel, or through the back passage to inspect the large bowel.

A *colonoscope* is the name give to the latter. From the outside a colonoscope is a flexible tube about 15mm wide and 1.5m long. At its front end are a lens, a bright light source and a small open channel through which specially designed instruments can be passed up from the base. Through other channels water and air can be gently pumped in and out of the bowel to clear the view. At the base of the colonoscope are control handles that operate cables running the length of the instrument. By adjusting the controls the curve of the colonoscope can be altered, particularly at the tip, which allows it to be guided around the bowel. The original design of colonoscope used a tightly packed bundle of flexible light-conducting fibres to take the image produced by the lens at the front and conduct it down to the eyepiece at the base. The most modern designs in fact use a tiny video camera at the tip to send the image electronically down the colonoscope and on to be magnified and displayed on a television screen to the side of the patient. This is more comfortable for the operator and allows many people to see the image simultaneously. By looking at the television display the doctor can see the internal lining of the bowel, and by altering the controls he or she can change the direction of view or home in on an area that needs closer inspection.

The optical quality and flexibility of modern colonoscopes is very high and in the hands of a trained 'endoscopist' a very detailed inspection of the bowel can be carried out.

A shorter version of the colonoscope, which is easier to use and allows inspection of the rectum and left side of the colon (which is where the majority of bowel cancers arise) is called a flexible sigmoidoscope. (The 'sigmoid' part of the colon is the lower part and gets its name because it is S-shaped.) As many people with possible IBS who are referred to a specialist for investigation will undergo colonoscopy (or sigmoidoscopy) it is described next in some more detail and is illustrated in figure 6.

COLONOSCOPY PROCEDURE
To get a clear view of the bowel it is obviously necessary for it to be cleared of faeces, so the preparation for a colonoscopy involves two or three days on a low-residue diet (one with little fibre or roughage) plus a fairly thorough laxative regime. Preparation for flexible sigmoidoscopy can be a bit less intensive.

The procedure itself is far less uncomfortable in practice than most people expect before it is done. A mild short-acting sedative drug is usually used just before the colonoscopy to help relax the patient, and this can be combined

Figure 6: Colonoscopy

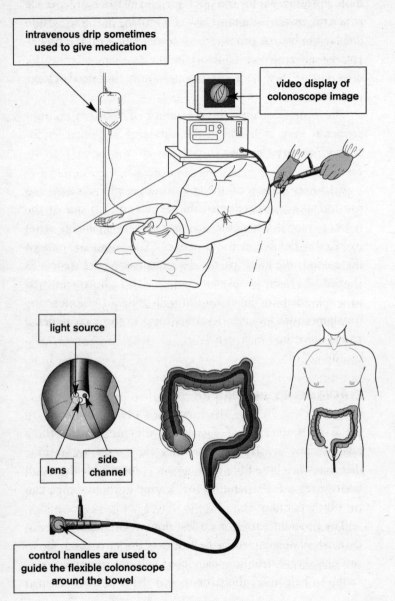

with a painkiller if necessary. The patient lies on his or her side and then the colonoscope is lubricated and gently advanced through the back passage and along the colon. A full colonoscopy can take about 20 minutes but sigmoidoscopy is quicker. The sedative wears off quickly and the patient can go home a short time later.

X-RAY (BARIUM ENEMA)

Until fibre-optic instruments came along X-ray examination was the only method available to show the interior structure of the complete bowel. It is still a very useful and widely used test, capable of showing even quite small details and it can be used in place of colonoscopy to investigate abdominal symptoms quite adequately. Modern digital machines use much less X-ray radiation than older models and the procedure is both safe and well tolerated.

When a photographic plate sensitive to X-rays is exposed to them it becomes darker (after development). Unlike visible light, X-rays can pass completely through the body but the extent varies according to the density of the particular tissue involved. Bones and teeth are the densest tissues and show up white on X-rays. Gas offers the least resistance and shows up dark on X-rays. To picture the bowel a technique is used in which a liquid ('barium') is used to coat the bowel lining, which is then slightly inflated with extra air. Barium is dense to X-rays and shows up white on the X-ray film. Because the bowel is filled out with air, which shows dark on the film, the resulting pictures can show the lining of the bowel quite well. Doctors refer to this air/barium technique as the 'double contrast' enema.

Barium enema examination requires the same sort of diet

and laxative preparation beforehand as colonoscopy. To carry out the procedure the patient lies down on the X-ray table, which is pretty much like an examination couch, underneath which are the X-ray plates. The X-ray tube is positioned above on a moveable mounting. Then a small tube is inserted into the patient's back passage and through this is run the barium mixture and some air. The barium mixture needs to coat the whole lining of the bowel, so there is a bit of rolling around required to ensure this happens effectively. The specialist (radiologist) uses television images to line up the X-ray pictures and a short time later the procedure is complete. Barium is completely harmless and is simply passed with the next few bowel movements.

The main disadvantage of the barium enema examination is that tissue samples cannot be obtained with it. It cannot see the same level of detail as colonoscopy, and the image is only in black and white, whereas a colonoscope provides a colour view of the bowel lining. Sometimes it is difficult to get good enough barium coating of the bowel to be able to see every part of it well. The S-shaped sigmoid colon can be the hardest region to visualise so double contrast barium enema is often combined with flexible sigmoidoscopy to get round this problem. A technically perfect barium enema, combined if necessary with sigmoidoscopy, is, however, very unlikely to miss detecting a bowel cancer.

The above tests are the main ones needed to check the bowel thoroughly, but are necessary in only a minority of people with IBS. If someone has a history of weight loss or anaemia then you will know by now that IBS is not the diagnosis anyway. Very often, though, the tests are done to be 'on the safe side' or reassure everyone – patient and doctor alike – that IBS is the problem and nothing else. This is by far the commonest reason for doing such tests, so one need not assume, if a specialist says you should have a colonoscopy or barium enema, that what they are not telling you is that they suspect a bowel cancer.

3. Patient factors

To be adequately reassured is a perfectly good reason to see a doctor and have tests done. A lot of the work a doctor does is not to make diagnoses of serious medical conditions but in fact to do the opposite and diagnose the absence of such disease. Following on from comments made in the last chapter about attitudes to IBS people can feel nervous about wanting to see a specialist. They do not want to appear 'neurotic' or 'obsessed with their health'. Some people feel uncomfortable asking to see a specialist, in case their GP takes this as some sort of criticism of his or her ability to make a diagnosis. This is very unlikely to be the case. A doctor who is good at picking up the clues from his or her patients will realise when a referral is the best way to allay any fears the patient may have, even if IBS does seem to be the reasonable explanation for the patient's trouble. The tests needed to confirm IBS are in any case outside the range of those available for a GP to directly request, so the help of a specialist is required if the diagnosis is at all in doubt. But rather than relying on the ability of your GP to deduce what's worrying you it's best to simply say if you'd feel better going for a consultant's opinion.

Some people may have raised anxiety about having a serious underlying bowel disorder if there is a strong family history of such conditions. Again, a good medical history should bring this to light but only a very small proportion of the population are truly at above average risk for bowel cancer or for inflammatory bowel disease (see page 48). If the worry is there, though, it will probably not go away just with the GP's reassurance and confirmatory tests should be done to dispel the anxiety.

4. Predominance of diarrhoea

Diarrhoea is defined as frequent bowel movements or the passage of abnormally soft or liquid stools. The range of normal bowel frequency and consistency in human beings is wide but a change from their normal habit is what takes people to the doctor. Some people have 'diarrhoea-predominant' IBS. Others have 'constipation-predominant' IBS and others get a bit of both.

When making a diagnosis in someone who seems in general to be describing IBS but in whom diarrhoea is predominant there are some alternative conditions that the doctor needs to consider:

PERSISTENT INFECTION
Some organisms that infect the gut can persist for a very long time afterwards. Samples of stool can be examined in the laboratory for this, although it may be necessary to send more than one specimen on different days. *Giardia* is a gut parasite present all over the world but is particularly common in the tropics and is picked up from contaminated water supplies. It is the commonest parasite imported back to the UK by tourists. (It also has the distinction of being the first organism from the gut to have been observed under

a microscope. The inventor of the microscope, Anton van Leeuwenhoek, observed *Giardia* in samples of his own stool in 1681!) Occasionally stool samples remain negative in people who have *Giardia* infection and then samples can be taken from the upper gut by endoscopy if there is a high degree of suspicion that this infection could be present. As treatment of *Giardia* is simple (a short course of antibiotics) and fairly effective many doctors simply give the treatment to a patient who has persistent diarrhoea after a return from the tropics and wait to see what happens.

LACTOSE INTOLERANCE

Lactose is the sugar present in milk. It is made of two types of sugar molecule – glucose and galactose – linked together and is indigestible in humans. To make it digestible the enzyme lactase, present in the lining of the small bowel, splits lactose into its component sugars, which are then absorbed. Lactase is present in the small bowel of infants but it declines in the adult population, particularly in Africans, Asians and South Americans in whom up to 90 per cent of adults may be lactase-deficient. In Northern Europeans lactase deficiency is less common, affecting only about 5 to 10 per cent of adults. In people who have lactase deficiency unabsorbed lactose gets through to the large bowel, where it is fermented by the bacteria present there. This can cause increased wind, abdominal pain and distension and diarrhoea.

Lactase deficiency does not always cause symptoms even in those people who have it, unless they take in enough lactose through milk and milk products to overload the gut's tolerance. Although a sophisticated medical test is available to detect lactose intolerance, a simple way to exclude it is to avoid dairy produce for two or three weeks – non-dairy milk is now widely available in supermarkets – and the symptoms should disappear. The importance of lactose intolerance should however not be overstated. It is not a major cause of diarrhoea and is no more common in people with IBS than in the general population.

COELIAC DISEASE

This is basically an allergic reaction against gluten – a protein present in wheat, rye and barley and which also may contaminate commercial oat flours. In people with this condition gluten triggers the gut immune system, leading to damage of the food-absorbing surface of the upper small bowel. Apart from diarrhoea, coeliac disease can lead to many other problems, including poor growth in children, weight loss, abdominal pain, vitamin deficiency and anaemia. Coeliac disease does not always cause symptoms and may remain undiagnosed throughout someone's life – 1 per cent of Northern Europeans may have coeliac disease but less than a tenth of these are recognised. Some people with 'IBS' probably have undiagnosed mild coeliac disease.

Treatment is with a gluten-free diet but unlike lactose withdrawal this is not something that can be done easily at home to show results in a short time. People with coeliac disease need to be seen and advised by a specialist in the condition. Diagnosing coeliac disease precisely requires samples to be taken from the upper small bowel for examination under the microscope but it is possible to carry out 'screening' tests on a blood sample very easily, and this can be done by a GP. Certain antibodies (called *antigliadin* and *antiendomysial* antibodies) are present in a high proportion of people with coeliac disease. Absence of these antibodies in a blood test makes coeliac disease unlikely. The treatment of coeliac disease is mainly to exclude gluten permanently from the diet.

BILE SALT MALABSORPTION

This is one of the rarer causes of diarrhoea, but it is worth bearing in mind as treatment can be very effective. Bile is a juice produced by the liver which flows into the digestive system in order to help digest fats. 'Bile salts' are the constituents of bile that aid digestion and they work a bit like detergents when doing the washing up, combining with fats in food in order to make them absorbable. Excess bile salts are usually re-absorbed from the lower small bowel and returned to the liver for re-use. This process can be inefficient for a variety of reasons, and if so, bile salts get through to the large bowel. Unfortunately, in the large bowel bile salts tend to be irritating and they have a laxative effect. Although a high-tech test exists that can measure whether bile salt malabsorption is present, there is a simple practical way of finding out. Colestyramine (Questran®) is a powder that can be taken by mouth and which binds to and renders harmless any excess bile salt lying in the gut. A dose of colestyramine daily will give results in a week or two if it works at all. Colestyramine is safe but is only available on prescription.

INFLAMMATORY BOWEL DISEASE

Inflammatory bowel disease refers to two conditions with some similarities in which the bowel lining becomes inflamed:

1. Ulcerative colitis (which affects only the lining of the large bowel)
2. Crohn's disease (which can cause inflammation anywhere in the digestive tract)

Ulcerative colitis (UC) causes ulceration and loss of the lining cells of the colon and rectum, although commonly it only involves a section, leaving the rest of the colon normal. Bloodstained diarrhoea is the classic symptom so it is unlikely to be confused with irritable bowel syndrome.

Crohn's disease can affect quite short sections of the digestive system and give symptoms very much like IBS. Unlike ulcerative colitis, Crohn's disease may not cause the loss of blood in the stools but it tends to narrow areas of the bowel where it is active, causing pain from partial obstruction of the bowel among other symptoms.

Clues to the presence of inflammatory bowel disease, apart from obvious ones like the passage of blood, will often be found in the blood tests done routinely in assessing IBS but occasionally inflammatory bowel disease comes to light only on full bowel examination.

OTHER CAUSES OF DIARRHOEA

Among the many other possible causes for regular diarrhoea are:

- Alcohol excess. Often this causes morning diarrhoea

- Drugs, such as non-steroidal anti-inflammatories (NSAIDs, like ibuprofen) are common culprits. Drugs to reduce heartburn (called proton pump inhibitors, like omeprazole) are another
- Bowel cancer
- Previous removal of the gall-bladder (cholecystectomy, 2–4 per cent of cases)

The preceding sections list the main alternative conditions that a doctor needs to exclude when seeing someone who presents with what appears to be IBS. However, when a good history, basic clinical examination and the simple blood tests all point to a diagnosis of IBS, it will almost always be correct.

Chapter 5

Treatment for IBS

One way of treating IBS is to randomly try different remedies until you find one that's helpful. Sometimes that works but it is inefficient and may miss the mark completely. It's possible to be a bit more logical in your approach. It pays to consider some points first:

Is any treatment necessary?

If the symptoms are mild and not too troublesome then all many people want to know is what's causing the problem, and that it is not too serious. Knowing that is enough for many to just get on and live with IBS.

Are there other non-bowel related issues?

Principally this means being honest about accompanying psychological problems. These might well be directly related to the IBS – for example, it could be that the symptoms have been so troublesome as to cause depression. More likely it will be hard to know which is the chicken and which the egg. Stress, an unsatisfactory personal relationship or work problems may all precipitate or worsen IBS, and if they get no attention, it is pretty likely that the IBS is not going to improve. IBS symptoms may be your body's way of telling you to slow down or to carry out some other sort of lifestyle maintenance.

Becoming informed about IBS

You are already doing this but knowing what it is that you are trying to overcome is an important part of succeeding. There are plenty of other sources of information and support concerning IBS, including the various support groups around the country. Although not everyone's cup of tea initially, it can be remarkably helpful to share your experiences with others. You'll find out that many other people from all walks of life get IBS, that they are just as sensible as you are and that some of the things they have found helpful in dealing with IBS might help you too. Some useful contacts are listed in appendix C.

Having realistic expectations

IBS treatment is not an easy off-the-shelf affair. Even if the treatment is well chosen to your own pattern of symptoms, you may find that the improvement is only partial. Sometimes the best you can do with IBS is to make it tolerable. It does not tend to go away.

General recommendations

Some actions are likely to be beneficial to everyone with IBS. These include cutting down on caffeine intake and reducing the amount of fat in the diet. Caffeine can stimulate the gut and the presence of fat in food triggers various reflex actions in the digestive system that amplify the symptoms of IBS. Regular exercise also helps. It's no coincidence that such manoeuvres also help make you feel healthier in general. Regular exercise is a good way to neutralise stress. Taking steps to improve your general well-being has a positive effect on most long-term medical conditions and improves your ability to cope with them.

Your IBS 'type'

For some of the luckier people who have IBS some lifestyle adjustment might be all they need to reduce their IBS to tolerable nuisance value, but most need to do more. To do this effectively it helps to have a strategy based on which of the three broad categories of IBS you have:

1 Mainly diarrhoea
2 Mainly constipation
3 Mainly pain (or bloating)

There is a large crossover among these groups and many people feel that their IBS flits between the three types, if not at the same time. Treatment strategies may therefore need to be flexible and fit in according to how your IBS is currently behaving.

Treating diarrhoea-predominant IBS

'Diarrhoea' is not a precise term and people vary a lot in what they mean by it. The range of 'normal' stool character and frequency is wide and what may be diarrhoea to one may be normal to another. A change from someone's normal bowel habit towards unduly loose or frequent stools covers the general definition. There is often some urgency involved, i.e. when you get the call to empty your bowel, you need to answer it in a hurry.

Diarrhoea in IBS tends not to be constant, i.e. the stools often veer towards being more firm again. Continuously loose stools are unlikely to be IBS, in which case a search for the rarer causes of diarrhoea is justified.

1. EXCLUDE RARE CAUSES OF DIARRHOEA

These were mentioned in the previous chapter. Gluten sensitivity (coeliac disease), persistent gut infection, lactose intolerance and bile salt malabsorption are uncommon causes of diarrhoea when the symptom picture otherwise looks like IBS, but it makes sense to exclude them. Blood antibody tests for coeliac disease are easily organised by the GP, as is stool analysis for infection. Lactose intolerance, causing diarrhoea related to dairy product intake, is less common in those of European racial origin but it is not very difficult to put yourself on a dairy produce-free diet for two or three weeks to test that possibility. Similarly it is easy to take colestyramine for a trial period. You can do yourself no harm by ticking these possibilities off the list.

Unless you are found to have one of these alternative bowel problems your next step is to check for any factors (food mainly) that could be triggering your IBS.

2. CHECK A FOOD DIARY

This does not need to be complicated, but it does need to be comprehensive. A careful note of all items eaten or drunk over two to three weeks, kept alongside a record of IBS symptoms, may show a previously unrecognised association. It is important to note everything taken. For example, sorbitol, an artificial sweetener widely used as a sugar substitute, can cause diarrhoea as can fructose, a common sugar. You will need to check the labels on the packaging to get such information.

Should your diary not reveal any obvious trigger foods you may wish to seriously consider an exclusion diet to detect less obvious problem foods. The pros, cons and practicalities of doing that are in chapter 7.

One point worth mentioning here but which is returned to in people with constipation-predominant IBS is the use of bran. 'Increase your bran intake' has become something of a mantra not only in IBS treatment but also as general health advice. Some people are, however, made worse by it. If you have been taking extra bran (or cereals containing extra fibre) in an attempt to help your IBS, it is possible it is having the reverse effect, so cut them out for a couple of weeks to check.

Like lactose avoidance, keeping a food diary might prove no help at all. It can be difficult to do or produce confusing results. Many specialists do not find food diaries helpful in managing their patients but if you are really bothered by your IBS you may wish to go through the process. It *can* be worthwhile.

3. USE 'ANTI-DIARRHOEA' MEDICINES
These are effective and helpful if properly used. They are not suitable for use in children.

a. Loperamide (Imodium®)
Loperamide acts fairly specifically on gut muscle to slow its activity and is commonly used to treat short-lived diarrhoea related to food poisoning and the like. In longer-term use it can give rise to cramping discomfort in the abdomen, which of course defeats the purpose of using it in IBS. However, if used cautiously and at the minimum effective dose, it is suitable for reducing diarrhoea, faecal urgency and incontinence. Each Loperamide capsule contains 2 milligrams (mg) of the drug. The maximum total dose in a day is 16mg, i.e. eight capsules, but one should aim to use less. As with any anti-diarrhoeal drug it is possible to take too much of it, and end up constipated. Small amounts of Loperamide can be bought without a prescription.

b. Codeine phosphate
Codeine is an opiate, i.e. a morphine-like drug, which can slow gut action and which also has pain-killing activity. It has the potential to become addictive, which is an important issue in a long-term condition like IBS. Codeine tablets come in 15mg and 30mg strengths and the dose is one or two at a time, up to four times daily. Codeine phosphate is a prescription-only drug.

Neither of these drugs is ideal for use on a regular basis. Loperamide does not have any addiction potential in regular use. They are most help in slowing bowel activity in advance of situations where it would be difficult or inconvenient to need to use the toilet in a hurry.

c. Serotonin (5-HT) blocking drugs

These drugs are relatively new and have a limited role in IBS. If you recall the information presented in chapter 2 about how nerves pass on signals, you will remember that certain chemical substances called neurotransmitters are involved in this process. Serotonin is one of these and was first discovered in the nineteenth century. In the mid twentieth century its chemical structure was identified, and its proper chemical name of 5-hydroxytryptamine applied. This is usually abbreviated to 5-HT.

5-HT has turned out to be an extremely important neurotransmitter for a variety of reasons. Ninety per cent of it in the body is concentrated in specialised cells within the lining of the gut but it is also present in blood and within the brain and nervous system. (For example, many modern antidepressant drugs and anti-migraine drugs work on 5-HT levels within the brain.)

In the gut 5-HT causes an increase in activity and this knowledge has spawned much interest in developing drugs that can alter the speed of gut action, based on whether they either block or boost the effects of 5-HT. Blocking 5-HT would tend to slow down gut activity and so would reduce diarrhoea. Conversely, a drug that boosted 5-HT in the gut would tend to relieve constipation.

Thus far the results of this research as far as IBS is concerned have been disappointing. A drug called alosetron, which blocks 5-HT (and so is called an 'antagonist') did show an improvement in diarrhoea in women with IBS, but it is associated with several side effects and is presently not available for prescription in the UK (the commonest side effect was constipation, but rarely some people experienced a serious type of bowel inflammation). Why it should be that only women got benefit from alosetron in this research is unknown. Further research into the use of 5-HT based drugs in IBS continues.

Treating constipation-predominant IBS

As with diarrhoea, defining constipation is not straightforward. One misconception is that constipation implies not moving your bowels every day. The range of normal bowel frequency in human beings can be up to once every three days, and a person who passes normal soft stools without any difficulty at this frequency, and always has done, is not constipated. If, however, someone gets a regular bowel action every day yet they always pass hard, dry, pellety stools like sheep droppings that cause discomfort all the time then they *are* constipated. The character of stool and the ease of getting rid of it can be more important than the frequency of bowel action. Truly constipated stools are the hard lumps just described.

People with IBS often get the urge to move their bowel and find themselves straining to get rid of it, yet if the stool that they consequently pass is soft and well formed then they have really been responding to the symptoms of their irritable bowel – in this case an irritable rectum (the 'reservoir' part of the lower bowel).

Hard, pellety stools occur when stools travel very slowly along the large bowel (i.e. there is a slow gut transit time). One of the functions of the large bowel is to extract water from the semi-liquid food residue that reaches it from the small bowel, and the longer the stool is in contact with the bowel wall the drier the stool becomes.

1. EXERCISE

Inactivity is associated with constipation, and taking some exercise regularly helps relieve constipation. People who exercise regularly also have a lower risk of getting bowel cancer, heart disease and diabetes.

2. FIBRE SUPPLEMENTS

Fibre tends to hold water and also provides extra stool bulk, which stimulates the 'moving along' muscles of the bowel (peristalsis), thus reducing transit time. The bulkier and softer stools also need less force from the gut muscles to be pushed along. Increasing dietary fibre is a natural consequence of eating more fruit and vegetables, which have a number of other health benefits too. Assuming, though, that you are already taking as much extra dietary fibre as you can manage then you can boost your intake with natural bran added to foods or with a range of fibre supplements, including those based on ispaghula husks (Fybogel®, Isogel®, Ispagel Orange® and Regulan) or on sterculia (Normacol®). All of the latter can be bought from a pharmacy but are also available on prescription.

The main problem with bran and fibre supplements is that they do not reliably help people with constipation-predominant IBS and they often make the symptoms of abdominal bloating and 'wind' worse. However, it is worth experimenting with small amounts infrequently at first and juggling around with the amount taken. Just enough may help relieve the constipation without worsening the other symptoms.

3. OSMOTIC LAXATIVES

Osmosis is the process by which fluids move across a membrane. Osmotic laxatives are liquid preparations taken by mouth which are not absorbed by the digestive system. Their presence in stools draws water back out of the bowel wall and into the stools, thus softening them. The two in common use are lactulose, a type of sugar (Regulose®, Duphulac®, Lactugal®), and macrogols (polyethylene glycols) such as Movicol®. A good fluid intake helps these types of laxative to work – lactulose comes as a syrup and macrogols as a powder that must be dissolved first in water. Lactulose commonly exacerbates bloating and borborygmi in people with IBS, so most specialists recommend Movical® instead.

4. STIMULANT LAXATIVES

Stimulant laxatives such as senna and bisacodyl work directly on the bowel to increase the activity of the gut muscles. Senna is a good and safe laxative and earlier worries that long-term use 'weakened' the bowel are no longer a concern. Many stimulant laxatives are obtainable across the counter in pharmacies and health food shops, some of which have pretty drastic effects. It is best to check with a pharmacist before trying any yourself. Remember also that when constipation starts happening it needs to be explained as well as treated, so check with your doctor if it occurs as a new symptom.

5. OTHER AGENTS
Tegaserod is a drug that boosts the effect of 5-HT in the bowel. It has been shown to relieve constipation in women with IBS but does not presently have a licence for use in the UK.

Treating abdominal pain and bloating

The third 'type' of IBS is that in which abdominal pain and bloating are the most troublesome symptoms.

1. 'ANTI-SPASM' DRUGS
It used to be thought that excessive activity of the gut wall muscles, leading to their spasm, was one of the main ways in which IBS arose. There is probably still some truth in the concept, although earlier sections of the book have mentioned that the perception of abdominal pain is more complicated than this. Drugs that reduce the strength of contraction of gut muscles are still widely used in IBS and can be helpful in some individuals. The evidence for their general effectiveness is, however, now recognised to be lacking, despite the fact that they continue to be widely prescribed for IBS.

There are two groups of gut spasm-reducing drugs:

1 Those that act directly on the smooth muscle of the gut.

These have few side effects.
2 Those that act on the nervous system of the gut. These tend to have side effects related to unwanted interference with the nervous system elsewhere in the body.

Direct gut smooth muscle relaxants
Mebeverine (Colofac®) and alverine (Spasmonal®) are two very similar drugs that can be taken between one and three times daily. Fybogel Mebeverine® is a brand combining mebeverine with ispaghula husk fibre supplement.

Peppermint oil (Colpermin®, Mintec®) is taken by mouth in capsules that dissolve sufficiently slowly so that the oil reaches the large bowel before being released. The capsules need to be swallowed whole as the oil is irritating to the mouth and upper digestive system.

All these medicines are available in over-the-counter preparations as well as being prescribable.

Other antispasmodic drugs
These block the action of a type of neurotransmitter in the general nervous system as well as in the gut. The former effect is undesirable but unavoidable, and as a result these drugs can cause side effects such as blurred vision, dry mouth, difficulty in passing urine and constipation. They can also worsen an eye condition called glaucoma, so are unsuitable for many, particularly older people with IBS.

Although there are several drugs in this group, the only two in common use for IBS are dicycloverine (Merbentyl®) and hyoscine (Buscopan®). They are both available with or without a prescription. Although individuals may feel that they do benefit from 'anti-spasm' drugs the results of research trials indicate that the 'placebo effect' of using them in IBS is so high that it is indistinguishable from the effects of the drugs.

2. ANTIDEPRESSANT DRUGS

There is evidence from several research studies that several types of 'older generation' antidepressant drugs can reduce abdominal pain in IBS. Amitriptyline is the most commonly used of these drugs, nortriptyline is another. The starting dose employed for IBS is less than that normally needed in treating depression. Low-dose antidepressants are quite frequently used in conditions that cause long-term pain and may work by reducing the transmission of pain 'signals' to the brain. Some of the positive results could also be from a small mood-enhancing effect too. Antidepressants are mainly of use in treating abdominal pain and diarrhoea in IBS. At higher doses these drugs tend to worsen constipation, so people with constipation-predominant IBS are the least likely to get any benefit from them.

Of the many difficulties that exist in treating IBS the lack of a wide range of effective medicines to choose from is one of the biggest problems. Many of the research trials examining the effectiveness of what is available have not been very well done, so the amount of evidence in favour of any one drug is poor compared to many other medical conditions. This may not matter so much to the individual, who will in any case probably wish to try several treatments to find out which works best for them, but there is clearly a need for a lot more choice. Given the numbers of likely customers, new effective, safe and well-tolerated IBS treatments will confidently ensure the financial future of their discoverer and there is indeed a lot of research activity in IBS by pharmaceutical companies. Several drugs are under evaluation and will hopefully show positive results within the next few years.

Psychological therapy

Psychological treatment is available through the NHS and is carried out by clinical psychologists, who are essentially experts in human behaviour and how to modify it. The sorts of methods psychologists use can take many forms, from teaching relaxation techniques to changing one's reactions to feeling or to stress. GPs can refer their patients directly to a clinical psychologist but in almost all areas of the country waiting lists for such services are long. Psychological methods have been used to treat IBS symptoms for nearly 40 years. The people with IBS most likely to respond favourably are those who are below 50 years old, whose symptoms are worse with stress, who have low levels of anxiety and who are not affected by long-term abdominal pain.

One of the barriers to considering psychological treatment is that many people wrongly consider it to be the sort of treatment that gets used only for 'illnesses of the mind' (implying such illnesses are less real or less valid than some other sorts). In fact, our response to any illness can be profoundly influenced for the good or bad by our individual psychological approach. Sometimes this can lead to the reinforcement of negative ideas and the worsening of symptoms. No matter what the nature of the illness it can be worthwhile learning how better to cope with it, and a clinical psychologist is the best person to teach this.

Chapter 6

Complementary Medicine for IBS

Interest in 'complementary' or 'alternative' treatments continues to grow rapidly in all areas of medicine, including IBS. Conventional drugs are often seen as working *against* natural processes (*anti*-diarrhoeal, *anti*-spasmodic) whereas complementary remedies are perceived as promoting balance and harmony, often on the grounds that are not very solidly based on conventional science.

To go deeply into this subject would take us into another book but one major advantage the pharmaceutical industry has over complementary medicine is the ability to fund studies that show that its products have an effect. Modern research trials cost sums of money that are out of the reach of most complementary treatments. The result is a body of literature on non-drug treatments that is puny compared to the output of the drug industry. We should not have different standards for assessing conventional and complementary treatments – all need to be rigorously scrutinised. The reality is that only a few complementary treatments can be fairly discussed in a book such as this, which attempts to provide the reader with a digest of current medical opinion. Despite the great popularity of complementary medical treatments, the quality of research undertaken on the majority does not compare to that undertaken with many pharmaceuticals.

Additional problems with things like herbal preparations arise from the variable amount of active (or potentially active) substance within them. Pharmaceutical products are rigorously controlled for quality and dosage whereas natural products may vary markedly in their content from batch to batch. Whereas the track record of production of a licensed drug provided by a qualified pharmacist in the UK will be completely reliable the same cannot be said of many products sold in health stores or other outlets.

Hypnotherapy

Hypnotherapy attempts to give people some control of normally subconscious body functions such as gut activity. Although demanding of therapy time, expensive and not generally available, there is good evidence to suggest that some people with IBS respond well to hypnotherapy, and that their improvement is maintained for a long time afterwards. In one major study in the UK 71 per cent of the group of IBS patients who initially responded to hypnotherapy maintained their improvement up to six years later.

Chinese herbal medicines

These are still used routinely in China for IBS, as they have probably been for centuries. Several Chinese studies have indicated their effectiveness, although the study methods were unsatisfactory from a Western scientific standpoint. However, one well-conducted research trial on Chinese herbal treatment for IBS carried out in Australia has shown very favourable results. Chinese medicine is usually individually tailored to the patient and may need to be modified as time goes by. The researchers studied the effect of such individualised treatment versus a standard treatment containing 20 Chinese herbs and compared these with a dummy treatment (placebo). Those patients receiving either the standard mixture or individualised treatments with herbs had about twice the improvement of the placebo group, the best results actually being with the standard mixture. This study has suggested that Chinese herbal medicine is a serious potential treatment choice for IBS.

Padma lax

This is a Tibetan herbal formula of 13 constituents that has been available in Switzerland for over 30 years as a remedy for constipation. In a study evaluating its effectiveness in constipation-predominant IBS it significantly improved constipation, abdominal pain and general IBS symptoms after three months. Loose stools occurred in some patients so it is probably not suitable for people who experience diarrhoea from IBS.

Artichoke leaf extract

A patented formulation of artichoke leaf extract, called Hepar-SL, given as capsules in a short trial of six weeks, was reported to improve abdominal pain, bloating or constipation in 84 per cent of those who took part.

Probiotics

Probiotics are microorganisms (such as bacteria) that are intended to be beneficial to health. Other than in well-recognised gut infections the basic idea that changes in the population of microorganisms within the gut are linked to many types of ill health is little more than speculation. For some years the concept of overgrowth of yeast (particularly *Candida*) within the gut has been put forward as an explanation not only for IBS but also for fatigue, headaches and many other disorders. Whereas the evidence in support of the 'candidiasis' theory has been weak at best the fact that many people who then undertook dietary changes to reduce the supposed gut overload of yeast then felt a lot better should not be discounted. It may well be that subtle changes to gut microorganism populations do help some people. Or it may be that some other part of the dietary change was actually what helped (including the placebo effect) – the jury is still out.

Evidence that deliberately changing gut bacterial populations is good, bad or indifferent is so far inconclusive. Some researchers also feel that the safety of probiotics is not yet well enough understood. The sort of probiotic products you can now buy easily in supermarkets are safe enough, but are untested as far as IBS is concerned (in fact how many live bacteria they actually contain after several weeks on the shelf is debatable too). At the moment it is not possible to make any recommendations concerning probiotics for IBS or any other condition.

Other complementary treatments

Homoeopathy is one of the most popular of complementary treatments and has been an integral part of available treatments since the inception of the NHS. Based on the principle of 'like cures like', dilute substances are chosen to match the patient's symptoms as much as possible. No sufficiently controlled studies on homoeopathy in IBS have been done, so its effectiveness in this condition remains untested.

Small trials of the use of acupuncture and of reflexology have shown no benefits of either in IBS.

Chapter 7

Food Intolerance, Allergy and IBS

General immune system reactions

Food undoubtedly has the capacity to cause undesired effects, and in a number of different ways. In a small proportion of the population who have 'classical' food allergy the ingestion of a small amount of the offending food will cause symptoms within minutes. The most extreme example of such reactions is one in which the tissues of the mouth, throat and upper airway can suddenly become swollen. This condition can be so severe as to be life-threatening. Peanuts are perhaps the best-known food associated with such reactions but the proportion of the population who are this sensitive is very small indeed.

Although rare, the process that goes on in these very obvious allergic reactions is quite well understood. The types of immune system cell involved are known, the chemicals these cells release upon meeting the food trigger and the effects these chemicals go on to have in the body are well recognised. Medical science does not have an issue with accepting and explaining this type of food allergy, and people who have this tendency don't usually need much help in detecting what the foods are that they need to avoid.

The immune system is known to react at different 'speeds', one could say, and the above example is of a food allergy that involves the fast-track system. A similarly quick allergic response is seen when you brush against stinging nettles and weals rise up on your skin within minutes. Or if you are allergic to cats and come into contact with one, you may well find yourself sneezing moments later.

The immune system also has a much slower system of response within its normal range of reactions. Vaccinations against infectious disease are an example, in which your immunity builds up over weeks following the injection and can be reinforced by a booster given months or even years later. All of this is standard textbook stuff, and there is no disagreement about it.

IBS and allergy

IBS, by definition almost, is not food allergy in the same sense as peanut sensitivity or nettle rash. In people with IBS no abnormalities are found within the immune system of the gut that can explain the symptoms. This might of course reflect the fact that our tests are too crude or that we simply do not yet understand the process going on – a healthy scepticism of one's level of knowledge is always a good thing in medical science. But in the absence of findings linking the immune system's function with the symptoms, using the term food *allergy* in connection with IBS is not generally useful.

Food intolerance

Food intolerance is a much wider concept than allergy and is within everyone's experience to some extent. A Chinese meal overloaded with monosodium glutamate to 'enhance' the taste will give a lot of people a headache. Red wine and cheese may trigger migraine in many people. The biology of what actually goes on in the body in such reactions is not very well understood, yet no one denies that such reactions exist. Whether intolerance to food can cause IBS symptoms is much more open to debate, but certainly for some people the answer is yes. Many studies have shown that a significant proportion of people who undertake some sort of dietary change along the lines of eliminating foods to which they seem intolerant will improve their IBS. The responses tend, however, to be individual and generalisations are almost impossible. What follows is a guide to a sensible approach to this topic, but it cannot be said to be based on a large amount of solid scientific research.

Incidentally, some of the more extreme devotees of the food intolerance (or allergy) camp get annoyed by what they see as the closed thinking of conventional medical research to their methods. Medicine does usually deserve its reputation for being conservative and a bit slow to adopt entirely new ways of thinking about illness but even the most broad-minded of medical scientists could be forgiven for doubting the validity of diagnosing and treating allergies of any type from clippings of hair, tests of skin electrical resistance or of some of the other types of test now so readily available. Should a reliable and safe treatment for IBS come along, then, no matter how unconventional, doctors will welcome it as much as any other group.

DETECTING FOOD INTOLERANCE

The relationship between a food to which you might be intolerant and the symptoms it may cause is not so helpfully immediate as it is with the fast-track immune response mentioned above. Furthermore, the culprit food might be something that you have been used to taking for years and if so you would be unlikely to suspect it. If your IBS tends only to cause constipation, it may not in any case be worth embarking on a quest for food intolerance. Such benefit as may be had is usually limited to people who get diarrhoea or abdominal discomfort, or both.

Elimination diets

The only way to find out in practical terms whether something you are eating is causing any symptoms is to eliminate it, when you should get better, and then re-introduce it, when you should get worse. But if you are intolerant of more than one food and don't eliminate both at the same time, you will fail to detect either of them. And if it is not so much a food but a component of food that might be present in a wide range of products that is the problem, then you have little chance of ever making sense of this issue. Cutting out single items, such as bread, is therefore the easiest way to go about food elimination but it is also the method with the least chance of success. Having said that, its big advantage is that it is feasible without the major commitment and potential disruption that more restricted diets entail.

You can therefore initially see if cutting out wheat, cereals, milk and eggs, while allowing yourself most vegetables, fruits, fish and meats, makes any difference. If so, then reintroduce a food group one at a time. Along with this simple restriction you can also cut out caffeine (tea, coffee, cola), chocolate and alcohol, all of which are foods that have some degree of 'chemical' effect on the body. Avoiding high-sugar and high-fat foods is also helpful.

If despite all these changes you are no better, if your IBS is really bothering you and you seriously want to be sure if it's food intolerance that's the cause of it then you need to go the whole hog.

EXCLUDING FOODS

The first phase of an elimination diet is one in which you convert to taking a very restricted diet for at least a week or two. This is the exclusion phase. Although the most drastic form of exclusion is fasting, this is not be recommended. Not only is it potentially unsafe but also your body will automatically go into fasting mode, which will itself generate symptoms. So forget that idea. You could go on to one of the very restricted diets that have historically been used, such as 'lamb and pears' or 'turkey and pears' – which are exactly what they sound like. If you can stand the boredom you will come to no nutritional harm from such a diet provided you are otherwise in good health, but remember that other medical conditions such as diabetes may make any sort of drastic dietary change problematic. Should you have any doubts then check first with your GP, who could also refer you to a dietician for more expert advice.

A practical alternative to very restricted diets like these is to go on to a 'few foods' or 'rare foods' exclusion diet. We now have so many different types of food available from around the world that it is not too difficult to put yourself on to a regime that contains foods you would ordinarily hardly ever eat. You will know what they might be, but for example less commonly used or exotic vegetables such as parsnips or yams, different types of grains and seeds like buckwheat, along with fresh meat, avoiding preserved or tinned produce and any types of flavourings or sauces could be put together in recipes that would be a substantial change from your usual. If during a couple of weeks or so on this you notice not the slightest bit of difference in your IBS symptoms then you are probably not food intolerant anyway.

If you notice a change for the better then you need slowly to re-introduce items, hesitating a few days to a week at each stage. Remember that in food intolerance the amount of a problem food may be quite important, with smaller amounts being tolerable.

More details on elimination diets can be had from a number of books written on this topic, one of which is listed in appendix A.

Conclusions

Irritable bowel syndrome is a group of common disorders of gut function. Although not serious, it can cause much disability. It occurs in the absence of currently detectable abnormalities of the gut and its causes are unknown. It can affect people of almost all ages and from any background. Broadly speaking it has three symptom patterns, which are mainly diarrhoea, mainly constipation or mainly abdominal pain, but combinations of symptoms are very common.

Adverse reactions to food are identifiable in only a minority of people with IBS, many of whom do not even consult a doctor about their symptoms. Treatment of IBS by dietary means or by medication has variable success and some people with IBS still find it causes them much bother no matter what they do. Unproven methods of treatment tend to proliferate when conventional medical treatment has failed to come up with the answers, and this is true of IBS.

Research into IBS is intensive and some lines of research are quite promising. Hopefully these will turn into useful treatments in the near future.

Appendix A

References

- Kennedy, T.M., et al., 'Irritable bowel syndrome' (Clinical Evidence, 2004; 11: 615–25); www.clinicalevidence.com/ceweb/conditions/dsd/0410/0410.jsp
- Talley, N.J., and Spiller, S., 'Irritable bowel syndrome: a little understood organic bowel disease?' (The Lancet, 2002; 360: 555–64); www.thelancet.com
- Rome Criteria for IBS: www.romecriteria.org
- Metz, H.R., 'Drug therapy: irritable bowel syndrome' (New England Journal of Medicine, 2003; 349(22): 2136–46); http://content.nejm.org/
- Thielecke, F., et al., 'Update in the pharmaceutical therapy of the irritable bowel syndrome' (International Journal of Clinical Practice, 2004; 58(4): 374–81).

- Cash, B.D., and Chey, W.D., 'Advances in the management of irritable bowel syndrome' (Current Gastroenterology Reports, 2003; 5: 468–75); www.current-reports.com
- Somers, S.C., and Lembo, A., 'Irritable bowel syndrome: evaluation and treatment' (Gastroenterology Clinics, June 2003; 32(2)).
- Bassotti, G., et al., 'Pharmacological treatment of irritable bowel syndrome: a critical assessment' (Scandinavian Journal of Gastroenterology, 2003; 10: 1013–15).
- Viera, A.J., et al., 'Management of irritable bowel syndrome' (American Family Physician, 2002; 66(10): 1867–74).
- Bensoussan A., et al., 'Treatment of irritable bowel syndrome with Chinese herbal medicine' (Journal of the American Medical Association, 1998; 280: 1585–89); http://jama.ama-assn.org/cgi/content/abstract/280/18/1585
- Kiefer, D., and Ali-Akbarian, L., 'A brief evidence-based review of two gastrointestinal illnesses: irritable bowel syndrome and leaky gut syndromes' (Alternative Therapies in Health and Medicine, 2004; 10(3): 22–30).
- Spannier, J.A., et al., 'A systematic review of alternative therapies in the irritable bowel syndrome' (Archives of Internal Medicine, 2003; 163: 265–74); http://archinte.ama-assn.org/cgi/content/abstract/163/3/265

Elimination diets

- Brostoff, Professor J., and Gamlin, L., *The Complete Guide to Food Allergy and Intolerance* (Bloomsbury, 1998).

Appendix B

Medication for IBS

The following information contains selected details of some of the medications used in treating irritable bowel syndrome. Full details are included in the manufacturer's data sheets and can also be viewed within the medicines section of the NetDoctor website: http://www.netdoctor.co.uk/medicines/

The information is accurate at the time of writing but new information on medicines appears regularly. A health professional should always be consulted concerning the prescription and use of medicines.

Medicines and their possible side effects can affect individual people in different ways. The following lists some of the side effects that are known to be associated with these medicines. Side effects other than those listed may exist.

1. Reduction of diarrhoea

LOPERAMIDE
Loperamide works by slowing the muscular contractions of the intestine. It does so by acting on special nerve receptors, called opioid receptors, which are found in the muscle lining the walls of the intestines. By acting on these receptors, loperamide reduces the muscular contractions of the intestine (peristalsis) that move food and faecal matter through the gut. Loperamide is usually used to treat short-term diarrhoea such as that caused by temporary gut infection. It can also be used to control chronic (long-term) diarrhoea, such as may occur in irritable bowel syndrome, on the advice of a doctor.

Main possible side effects
- Excessive slowing of gut activity
- Abdominal cramps
- Dry mouth
- Drowsiness
- Fatigue
- Dizziness
- Nausea and vomiting
- Bloating
- Skin reactions such as rash and itch

Other medicines containing the same active ingredient
Arret, Diah-limit, Diaquitte, Diocalm ultra, Entrocalm, Imodium, Normaloe, Nucare loperamide

2. Reduction of abdominal pain

MEBEVERINE
Mebeverine acts directly on the smooth muscle in the gut, causing it to relax. It also prevents nerve signals getting through to the muscle in the intestines. This also causes the muscle to relax, preventing painful muscle spasm.

Main possible side effects
Mebeverine is usually well tolerated, but possible side effects include:

- Constipation
- Confusion
- Agitation

Other medicines containing the same active ingredients
Colofac 100, Colofac IBS, Colofac MR, Equilon, Fomac

DICYCLOVERINE
Dicycloverine hydrochloride (previously called dicyclomine hydrochloride in the UK) is a type of medicine called an anticholinergic. It works by relaxing the involuntary muscle found in the walls of the stomach and intestines (gastro-intestinal tract).

It does this by blocking nerve receptors called cholinergic (or muscarinic) receptors that are found on the surface of the muscle cells. This prevents a chemical called acetylcholine from acting on these receptors. Acetylcholine acting on these receptors normally causes the muscle to contract. By reducing this, dicycloverine helps the muscle in the digestive tract to relax.

Main possible side effects
Cholinergic nerve receptors are found widely in the body, not just the digestive system. Drugs such as dicycloverine can therefore have a wide range of side effects but at the doses used for irritable bowel syndrome these tend not to be common.

- Dry mouth
- Headache
- Constipation
- Blurred vision
- Difficulty in passing urine (urinary retention)
- Confusion

Other medicines containing the same active ingredients
Merbentyl, Merbentyl 20

AMITRIPTYLINE
Amitriptyline is a type of antidepressant. In smaller doses than usually needed for depression many antidepressants can alleviate pain. Amitriptyline can be effective in IBS.

Main possible side effects
These are similar to dicycloverine, as amitriptyline also blocks cholinergic nerve receptors. At the low doses used in IBS they tend not to be troublesome.

- Constipation
- Blurred vision
- Dry mouth
- Difficulty in passing urine (urinary retention)

- Drowsiness
- Confusion
- Sweating
- Blood disorders (rare)
- Disturbances of the gut such as diarrhoea, constipation, nausea, vomiting or abdominal pain
- Low blood pressure

Appendix C

Useful Contacts

Irritable Bowel Syndrome Network

Provides information and support for people with IBS, including details of local support groups and a helpline.

IBS Network
Northern General Hospital
Sheffield
S5 7AU
Tel: 0114 261 1531
Fax: 0114 261 0112
Email: info@ibsnetwork.org.uk

HELPLINE
IBS Network Helpline: 01543 492 192
(Open every weekday evening from 18.00 to 20.00 and on Saturday mornings from 10.00 to 12.00.)

Digestive Disorders Foundation

A national charity covering the entire range of digestive disorders. (It intends changing its name to Core during 2004.) Provides information for the public and funds research in these conditions. Information factsheets are available online or by post (include SAE) from:

Digestive Disorders Foundation
PO Box 251
Edgware
Middlesex
HA8 6HG
Email: ddf@digestivedisorders.org.uk

For research and other enquiries:
Digestive Disorders Foundation
3 St Andrew's Place
London NW1 4LB

Tel: 020 7486 0341
Fax: 020 7224 2012